THE BODY BLUEPRINT

A Complete Guide to Understanding Your Inner Self

Decoding Your Body's Signals: Hormones, Fluids, Systems, and
Tests for Optimal Health

Disclaimer

The information contained in this book, "The Body Blueprint," is intended for general knowledge and informational purposes only and does not constitute medical advice.

This book is not intended to diagnose, treat, cure, or prevent any disease or medical condition. The content presented herein should not be used as a substitute for professional medical advice, diagnosis, or treatment. Always consult with a qualified healthcare professional, such as a physician or other licensed healthcare provider, for any health concerns, medical conditions, or before making any decisions related to your health or treatment. The author and publisher make no representations or warranties of any kind, express or implied, about the completeness, accuracy, reliability, suitability, or availability with respect to the information contained in this book for any purpose.

Any reliance you place on such information is therefore strictly at your own risk. The author and publisher shall not be held liable for any loss or damage, including without limitation, indirect or consequential loss or damage, or any loss or damage whatsoever arising from loss of *data* or profits arising out of, or in connection with, the use of this information.

Foreword

In a world increasingly focused on external appearances, it's easy to overlook the intricate and fascinating world within. Your body is a complex and finely tuned machine, a symphony of interconnected systems working tirelessly to keep you alive and thriving. This book, "The Body Blueprint," is your personal guide to understanding this remarkable inner landscape.

This isn't a medical textbook; it's a user-friendly manual designed to empower you with knowledge about your own body. From the elemental composition of your cells to the delicate balance of hormones, we'll explore the key components that make you, you. We'll delve into the vital roles of vitamins, minerals, proteins, and carbohydrates, and explain how their balance impacts your health. We'll also discuss common tests used to assess bodily functions, providing normal ranges and explaining what deviations might signify.

This book is for anyone who wants to take a proactive approach to their health and well-being. Whether you're a teenager just beginning to understand your body, an adult seeking to optimize your health, or simply someone curious about the inner workings of the human form, "The Body Blueprint" will provide you with the knowledge you need to become truly self-aware. By understanding your body's signals, you can make informed choices about your diet, lifestyle, and overall health, leading to a more vibrant and fulfilling life. Know thyself, for thy good.

Who Should Read This Book?

- Teenagers and young adults seeking to understand their developing bodies.
- Adults interested in optimizing their health and well-being.
- Individuals seeking to understand medical test results and their implications.
- Anyone interested in learning more about the human body and its functions.

How Will This Book Benefit You?

- Gain a comprehensive understanding of your body's systems and functions.
- Learn about the importance of nutrition and how it impacts your health.
- Understand common medical tests and their results.
- Become more self-aware and proactive about your health.
- Make informed decisions about your diet, lifestyle, and healthcare.

Table of Contents

Part 1

Chapter 1: The Human Body: An Overview

The human body is an extraordinary feat of biological engineering, a complex and intricately organized system of organs, tissues, and cells working in perfect harmony. This chapter provides a foundational overview of this remarkable structure, introducing the key levels of organization and the major organ systems that will be explored in greater detail throughout this book. Understanding this basic framework is essential for grasping how the body functions as a whole and how different parts contribute to overall health and well-being.

Levels of Organization:

The human body is organized hierarchically, with each level building upon the previous one:

- **Chemical Level:** This is the most basic level, encompassing atoms and molecules. Atoms, such as oxygen, carbon, hydrogen, and nitrogen, are the building blocks of all matter. These atoms combine to form molecules, such as water (H_2O), proteins, carbohydrates, lipids (fats), and nucleic acids (DNA and RNA). These molecules are essential for all bodily functions.
- **Cellular Level:** Cells are the fundamental units of life. They are the smallest structures capable of carrying out all the processes necessary for life. Cells vary greatly in size, shape, and function, but they all share some common characteristics, including a cell membrane, cytoplasm, and genetic material (DNA). Examples include blood cells, muscle cells, nerve cells, and bone cells.
- **Tissue Level:** Tissues are groups of similar cells that work together to perform a specific function. There are four primary types of tissues in the human body:

- **Epithelial Tissue:** Covers the body's surfaces, both internal and external. It forms protective barriers, lines organs and cavities, and is involved in secretion and absorption. Examples include the skin, the lining of the digestive tract, and the lining of blood vessels.
  - **Connective Tissue:** Provides support, structure, and connection for other tissues and organs. It includes various types of tissues, such as bone, cartilage, blood, and adipose (fat) tissue.
  - **Muscle Tissue:** Responsible for movement. There are three types of muscle tissue: skeletal muscle (responsible for voluntary movements), smooth muscle (found in the walls of internal organs), and cardiac muscle (found in the heart).
  - **Nervous Tissue:** Carries electrical signals throughout the body. It consists of nerve cells (neurons) and supporting cells (glia). Nervous tissue is responsible for coordinating and controlling bodily functions.
- **Organ Level:** An organ is a structure composed of two or more different types of tissues that work together to perform a specific function. The heart, for instance, is made up of muscle tissue (for contraction), connective tissue (for support), nervous tissue (for regulating heart rate), and epithelial tissue (lining the chambers). Other examples of organs include the brain, lungs, stomach, kidneys, liver, and skin.
- **Organ System Level:** An organ system is a group of organs that work together to perform a complex function necessary for survival. For example, the digestive system includes the mouth, esophagus, stomach, intestines, liver, and pancreas, all working together to digest and absorb nutrients from food.
- **Organismal Level:** This is the highest level of organization, representing the entire living being—the

human body—with all organ systems working together in a coordinated manner to maintain life.

The Major Organ Systems:

The human body consists of eleven major organ systems:

1. **Integumentary System:** Provides protection, regulates body temperature, and helps with sensory perception (skin, hair, nails).
2. **Skeletal System:** Provides support, structure, and protection for internal organs and enables movement (bones, cartilage, ligaments).
3. **Muscular System:** Enables movement, maintains posture, and generates heat (muscles).
4. **Nervous System:** Controls and coordinates bodily functions, transmits signals between different parts of the body, and is responsible for thought, memory, and emotions (brain, spinal cord, nerves).
5. **Endocrine System:** Regulates bodily functions through the release of hormones (glands such as the pituitary, thyroid, adrenal, and pancreas).
6. **Cardiovascular System:** Transports blood, oxygen, nutrients, and hormones throughout the body (heart, blood vessels).
7. **Lymphatic System:** Helps maintain fluid balance, defends against infection, and absorbs fats from the digestive system (lymph nodes, lymphatic vessels, spleen).
8. **Respiratory System:** Exchanges gases (oxygen and carbon dioxide) between the body and the environment (lungs, trachea, bronchi).
9. **Digestive System:** Breaks down food, absorbs nutrients, and eliminates waste (mouth, esophagus, stomach, intestines, liver, pancreas).

10. **Urinary System:** Filters waste from the blood and eliminates it from the body (kidneys, ureters, bladder, urethra).
11. **Reproductive System:** Responsible for reproduction (ovaries in females, testes in males).

In subsequent chapters, we'll dive deep into each of these systems, exploring their individual components and their interactions with other systems. This foundational understanding sets the stage for a comprehensive exploration of your "Body Blueprint."

Chapter 2: Elemental Composition: The Minerals That Make You

While we often visualize our bodies as organs and intricate systems, at a fundamental level, we are composed of chemical elements. These elements, particularly minerals, are the essential building blocks that contribute to numerous bodily functions, from forming strong bones and teeth to facilitating nerve impulses and regulating cellular processes. This chapter explores the key minerals that constitute the human body and their vital roles in maintaining health and well-being.

What are Minerals?

Minerals are naturally occurring inorganic substances that are essential for human health. Unlike vitamins, which are organic compounds, minerals are inorganic and retain their chemical structure. They are obtained through diet and play diverse roles in the body.

Major Minerals:

These minerals are required in relatively larger amounts (more than 100 milligrams per day).

- **Calcium (Ca):** The most abundant mineral in the body, with approximately 99% residing in bones and teeth, providing structural integrity. The remaining 1% circulates in the blood, performing crucial functions:
    - **Muscle Contraction:** Calcium ions trigger muscle contraction by interacting with muscle proteins.

- o **Nerve Transmission:** It facilitates the release of neurotransmitters, enabling communication between nerve cells.
  - o **Blood Clotting (Coagulation):** Calcium is a crucial component in the complex cascade of events that lead to blood clot formation, preventing excessive bleeding.
  - o **Cell Signaling:** It acts as a secondary messenger within cells, regulating various cellular processes.
  - o **Normal Range (Blood):** 8.5-10.5 mg/dL (milligrams per deciliter)
  - o **Below Normal (Hypocalcemia):** Can manifest as muscle cramps, spasms, numbness, tingling sensations, and in severe cases, seizures. Long-term deficiency increases the risk of osteoporosis (weak and brittle bones).
  - o **Above Normal (Hypercalcemia):** May lead to fatigue, muscle weakness, constipation, nausea, vomiting, and in severe instances, kidney stones and heart rhythm abnormalities.
- **Phosphorus (P):** The second most abundant mineral, with about 85% found in bones and teeth, working in conjunction with calcium to provide strength. The remaining phosphorus is involved in:
  - o **Energy Production (ATP):** A key component of ATP (adenosine triphosphate), the body's primary energy source.
  - o **DNA and RNA Formation:** A structural component of DNA and RNA, the carriers of genetic information.

- o **Cell Membrane Structure:** Forms part of phospholipids, the building blocks of cell membranes.
  - o **Acid-Base Balance:** Helps regulate the body's pH balance.
  - o **Normal Range (Blood):** 2.5-4.5 mg/dL
  - o **Below Normal (Hypophosphatemia):** Can result in muscle weakness, bone pain, fatigue, and in severe cases, respiratory difficulties.
  - o **Above Normal (Hyperphosphatemia):** Often observed in individuals with kidney disease and can contribute to calcium deposits in soft tissues.
- **Magnesium (Mg):** Participates in hundreds of biochemical reactions:
  - o **Muscle and Nerve Function:** Essential for muscle relaxation and proper nerve impulse transmission.
  - o **Blood Sugar Control:** Helps regulate blood glucose levels.
  - o **Blood Pressure Regulation:** Contributes to maintaining healthy blood pressure.
  - o **Bone Health:** Plays a role in bone strength and density.
  - o **Protein Synthesis:** Involved in the production of proteins.
  - o **Normal Range (Blood):** 1.7-2.2 mg/dL
  - o **Below Normal (Hypomagnesemia):** Can cause muscle cramps, tremors, weakness, fatigue, and heart rhythm irregularities.
  - o **Above Normal (Hypermagnesemia):** Relatively rare, typically occurring in individuals with impaired kidney function.

Can lead to muscle weakness, low blood pressure, and slowed breathing.
- **Sodium (Na):** A major electrolyte crucial for:
  - **Fluid Balance:** Helps regulate the distribution of water in the body.
  - **Nerve and Muscle Function:** Essential for nerve impulse transmission and muscle contraction.
  - **Blood Pressure Regulation:** Plays a role in maintaining blood pressure.
  - **Normal Range (Blood):** 135-145 mEq/L (milliequivalents per liter)
  - **Below Normal (Hyponatremia):** Can manifest as headache, nausea, vomiting, confusion, and in severe cases, seizures and coma.
  - **Above Normal (Hypernatremia):** May cause intense thirst, dehydration, confusion, and in severe cases, seizures and coma.
- **Potassium (K):** Another essential electrolyte:
  - **Muscle Contractions:** Particularly important for heart muscle function.
  - **Nerve Impulse Transmission:** Essential for nerve signaling.
  - **Fluid and Electrolyte Balance:** Helps maintain the proper balance of fluids and electrolytes in the body.
  - **Blood Pressure Regulation:** Contributes to maintaining healthy blood pressure.
  - **Normal Range (Blood):** 3.5-5.0 mEq/L
  - **Below Normal (Hypokalemia):** Can cause muscle weakness, cramps, constipation, heart rhythm abnormalities, and fatigue.

- o **Above Normal (Hyperkalemia):** Can be dangerous, potentially leading to life-threatening heart rhythm disturbances.

- **Chloride (Cl):** Often found in conjunction with sodium as sodium chloride (table salt), chloride is another essential electrolyte that plays a vital role in:
  - o **Fluid balance:** Chloride helps regulate fluid balance in the body, working alongside sodium.
  - o **Acid-base balance:** Chloride helps maintain the body's pH balance.
  - o **Digestion:** Chloride is a component of stomach acid (hydrochloric acid), which is essential for digestion.
  - o **Nerve impulse transmission:** Chloride is involved in nerve signaling.
  - o **Normal Range (Blood):** 95-105 mEq/L
  - o **Below Normal (Hypochloremia):** Can be caused by excessive vomiting, diarrhea, or certain medications. Symptoms can include dehydration, muscle weakness, and metabolic alkalosis (a condition where the body's pH becomes too alkaline).
  - o **Above Normal (Hyperchloremia):** Can be caused by dehydration, kidney disease, or certain medications. Symptoms can include dehydration, rapid breathing, and metabolic acidosis (a condition where the body's pH becomes too acidic).

Trace Minerals:

These minerals are required in much smaller amounts (less than 100 milligrams per day), but they are no less important for health.

- **Iron (Fe):** Iron is essential for:
    - **Oxygen transport:** Iron is a key component of hemoglobin, the protein in red blood cells that carries oxygen from the lungs to the rest of the body. It is also a component of myoglobin, which stores oxygen in muscles.
    - **Energy production:** Iron is involved in cellular respiration, the process by which cells produce energy.
    - **Immune function:** Iron plays a role in immune system function.
    - **Cognitive function:** Iron is important for brain development and cognitive function.
    - **Normal Range (Blood - varies by test, example: Serum Iron):** 60-170 mcg/dL (micrograms per deciliter)
    - **Below Normal (Iron Deficiency/Anemia):** Can lead to fatigue, weakness, shortness of breath, pale skin, and impaired cognitive function.
    - **Above Normal (Iron Overload/Hemochromatosis):** Can cause damage to organs such as the liver, heart, and pancreas.
- **Zinc (Zn):** Zinc is involved in numerous bodily functions, including:
    - **Immune function:** Zinc is essential for immune system function and wound healing.

- o **Cell growth and division:** Zinc is involved in cell growth, division, and DNA synthesis.
  - o **Enzyme activity:** Zinc is a cofactor for many enzymes, which are proteins that catalyze biochemical reactions.
  - o **Taste and smell:** Zinc is important for taste and smell perception.
  - o **Normal Range (Blood):** 70-120 mcg/dL
  - o **Below Normal (Zinc Deficiency):** Can cause impaired immune function, delayed wound healing, loss of taste and smell, and growth retardation in children.
  - o **Above Normal (Zinc Toxicity):** Can cause nausea, vomiting, diarrhea, and impaired immune function.
- **Copper (Cu):** Copper plays a role in:
  - o **Iron metabolism:** Copper is involved in iron absorption and transport.
  - o **Enzyme activity:** Copper is a cofactor for several enzymes, including those involved in energy production and antioxidant defense.
  - o **Nerve function:** Copper is important for nerve function.
  - o **Normal Range (Blood):** 70-140 mcg/dL
  - o **Below Normal (Copper Deficiency):** Can cause anemia, neurological problems, and impaired immune function.
  - o **Above Normal (Copper Toxicity):** Can cause nausea, vomiting, diarrhea, and liver damage.
- **Iodine (I):** Iodine is essential for:
  - o **Thyroid hormone production:** Iodine is a key component of thyroid hormones, which

regulate metabolism, growth, and development.
  - **Normal Range (Urine Iodine):** 100-200 mcg/L
  - **Below Normal (Iodine Deficiency):** Can lead to hypothyroidism (underactive thyroid), which can cause fatigue, weight gain, and impaired cognitive function. In pregnant women, iodine deficiency can cause developmental problems in the fetus.
  - **Above Normal (Iodine Excess):** Can also lead to thyroid problems, including hyperthyroidism (overactive thyroid).
- **Selenium (Se):** Selenium is a component of several enzymes, including:
  - **Antioxidant defense:** Selenium is a component of glutathione peroxidases, which are important antioxidant enzymes.
  - **Thyroid hormone metabolism:** Selenium is involved in the conversion of thyroid hormones.
  - **Immune function:** Selenium plays a role in immune system function.
  - **Normal Range (Blood):** 8-25 mcg/dL
  - **Below Normal (Selenium Deficiency):** Can increase the risk of certain cancers, heart disease, and thyroid problems.
  - **Above Normal (Selenium Toxicity):** Can cause hair loss, nail brittleness, and neurological problems.
- **Manganese (Mn):** Manganese is involved in:
  - **Bone formation:**
  - **Wound healing:**
  - **Metabolism:**

- o **Antioxidant defense:**
  - o **Normal Range (Blood):** 4-15 mcg/L
  - o **Below Normal (Manganese Deficiency):** Is rare but can affect bone health.
  - o **Above Normal (Manganese Toxicity):** Can cause neurological problems, particularly in individuals exposed to high levels of manganese in the environment.
- **Molybdenum (Mo):** Molybdenum is a cofactor for several enzymes involved in:
  - o **Metabolism:**
  - o **Waste product removal:**
  - o **Normal Range (Blood):** 0.4-1.1 mcg/L
  - o **Below Normal (Molybdenum Deficiency):** Is rare.
  - o **Above Normal (Molybdenum Toxicity):** Can cause gout-like symptoms.
- **Fluoride (F):** Fluoride is known for its role in:
  - o **Dental health:** Fluoride strengthens tooth enamel and helps prevent cavities.
  - o **Optimal Intake:** Varies based on age and source.
  - o **Below Normal (Fluoride Deficiency):** Increases the risk of dental cavities.
  - o **Above Normal (Fluoride Toxicity/Fluorosis):** Can cause dental fluorosis (discoloration of teeth) in children during tooth development and, in severe cases, skeletal fluorosis (affecting bones).

This completes the discussion of essential minerals. In the next chapter, we'll delve into the other crucial components of our diet: vitamins, proteins, and carbohydrates. Let me know when you're ready to proceed.

Chapter 3: Essential Nutrients: Vitamins, Minerals, Proteins, and Carbohydrates

Maintaining optimal health requires a balanced intake of essential nutrients. These nutrients are substances the body needs to function properly but cannot synthesize on its own, so we must obtain them through our diet. This chapter explores three key categories of nutrients: vitamins, proteins, and carbohydrates.

Vitamins:

Vitamins are organic compounds that are essential for various bodily functions. They are categorized as either water-soluble or fat-soluble.

- **Water-Soluble Vitamins:** These vitamins dissolve in water and are not stored in the body to a significant extent. Therefore, they need to be consumed regularly.
    - **Vitamin C (Ascorbic Acid):** Important for immune function, collagen synthesis (for skin, bones, and connective tissue), and antioxidant protection. Deficiency (Scurvy) can cause weakness, fatigue, bleeding gums, and impaired wound healing. Excess is usually excreted in urine.
    - **B Vitamins:** A group of eight vitamins that play crucial roles in energy metabolism, nerve function, and cell growth and division.
        - **B1 (Thiamine):** Important for energy metabolism and nerve function. Deficiency (Beriberi) can cause

neurological problems, muscle weakness, and heart problems.

- **B2 (Riboflavin):** Involved in energy metabolism and cell growth. Deficiency can cause skin problems, mouth sores, and eye issues.
- **B3 (Niacin):** Important for energy metabolism, DNA repair, and skin health. Deficiency (Pellagra) can cause skin problems, digestive issues, and neurological problems. High doses can cause flushing.
- **B5 (Pantothenic Acid):** Involved in energy metabolism and hormone production. Deficiency is rare.
- **B6 (Pyridoxine):** Important for protein metabolism, nerve function, and red blood cell formation. Deficiency can cause neurological problems, skin problems, and anemia.
- **B7 (Biotin):** Involved in carbohydrate, fat, and protein metabolism. Deficiency is rare.
- **B9 (Folate/Folic Acid):** Crucial for cell growth and division, especially during pregnancy. Deficiency can cause anemia and birth defects.
- **B12 (Cobalamin):** Important for nerve function, red blood cell formation, and DNA synthesis. Deficiency can cause anemia and neurological problems.

- **Fat-Soluble Vitamins:** These vitamins dissolve in fat and are stored in the body. Therefore, excessive intake can lead to toxicity.
  - **Vitamin A (Retinol):** Important for vision, immune function, cell growth, and reproduction. Deficiency can cause night blindness, impaired immune function, and skin problems. Excess can cause toxicity, leading to nausea, vomiting, and liver damage.
  - **Vitamin D (Calciferol):** Important for calcium absorption, bone health, and immune function. Deficiency can cause rickets in children and osteoporosis in adults. Excess can lead to hypercalcemia (high blood calcium).
  - **Vitamin E (Tocopherol):** An antioxidant that protects cells from damage. Deficiency is rare.
  - **Vitamin K (Phylloquinone/Menaquinone):** Essential for blood clotting. Deficiency can lead to bleeding problems.

Proteins:

Proteins are large molecules made up of amino acids. They are essential for building and repairing tissues, producing enzymes and hormones, and supporting immune function.

- **Amino Acids:** The building blocks of proteins. There are 20 amino acids, 9 of which are considered essential because the body cannot produce them and must obtain them from the diet.
- **Functions of Proteins:**

- o **Building and repairing tissues:** Muscles, skin, hair, and organs are made up of protein.
  - o **Enzyme production:** Enzymes are proteins that catalyze biochemical reactions.
  - o **Hormone production:** Many hormones are proteins.
  - o **Immune function:** Antibodies are proteins that help fight infection.
  - o **Transport:** Proteins transport nutrients and other substances throughout the body.
- **Protein Deficiency:** Can lead to muscle wasting, weakness, impaired immune function, and growth retardation in children.
- **Excess Protein:** While generally not harmful for healthy individuals in moderate amounts, very high protein intake over a long period can put a strain on the kidneys.

Carbohydrates:

Carbohydrates are the body's primary source of energy. They are classified as simple or complex.

- **Simple Carbohydrates (Sugars):** These are quickly digested and provide a rapid source of energy. Examples include glucose, fructose, and sucrose.
- **Complex Carbohydrates (Starches and Fiber):** These are digested more slowly and provide a sustained release of energy. Examples include whole grains, vegetables, and legumes.
- **Functions of Carbohydrates:**

- o **Energy source:** The primary source of energy for the body, especially the brain and nervous system.
  - o **Fiber:** Important for digestive health.
- **Carbohydrate Deficiency:** Can lead to fatigue, weakness, and difficulty concentrating.
- **Excess Carbohydrates (especially refined sugars):** Can contribute to weight gain, type 2 diabetes, and other health problems.

This detailed explanation of vitamins, proteins, and carbohydrates provides a comprehensive understanding of these essential nutrients. In the next chapter, we'll begin our deep dive into the body's systems, starting with the endocrine system. Let me know when you are ready to proceed.

Chapter 4: The Endocrine System: The Hormone Orchestrators

The endocrine system is a complex network of glands that produce and secrete hormones, chemical messengers that regulate a wide range of bodily functions. These functions include metabolism, growth and development, reproduction, mood, and sleep. Unlike the nervous system, which uses rapid electrical signals, the endocrine system uses slower, more sustained chemical signaling through the bloodstream.

What are Hormones?

Hormones are chemical substances produced by endocrine glands and released into the bloodstream. They travel to target cells or organs, where they bind to specific receptors and trigger a response. Hormones act as messengers, coordinating communication between different parts of the body.

Key Endocrine Glands and Their Hormones:

- **Hypothalamus:** Located in the brain, the hypothalamus acts as the control center of the endocrine system. It links the nervous system to the endocrine system and regulates the pituitary gland. It produces several releasing and inhibiting hormones that control the pituitary.
- **Pituitary Gland:** Often called the "master gland," the pituitary gland is located at the base of the brain and is controlled by the hypothalamus. It secretes several key hormones:

- o **Growth Hormone (GH):** Stimulates growth and cell reproduction.
  - o **Adrenocorticotropic Hormone (ACTH):** Stimulates the adrenal glands to produce cortisol.
  - o **Thyroid-Stimulating Hormone (TSH):** Stimulates the thyroid gland to produce thyroid hormones.
  - o **Follicle-Stimulating Hormone (FSH) and Luteinizing Hormone (LH):** Regulate reproductive functions.
  - o **Prolactin:** Stimulates milk production.
  - o **Antidiuretic Hormone (ADH):** Regulates water balance.
  - o **Oxytocin:** Involved in uterine contractions during childbirth and milk ejection.
- **Thyroid Gland:** Located in the neck, the thyroid gland produces thyroid hormones:
  - o **Thyroxine (T4) and Triiodothyronine (T3):** Regulate metabolism, growth, and development.
  - o **Normal Range (TSH):** 0.4-4.0 mIU/L (milli-international units per liter). T4 and T3 ranges vary by lab.
  - o **Below Normal TSH/High T4/T3 (Hyperthyroidism):** Can cause rapid heartbeat, weight loss, anxiety, and heat intolerance.
  - o **Above Normal TSH/Low T4/T3 (Hypothyroidism):** Can cause fatigue, weight gain, constipation, and cold intolerance.
- **Parathyroid Glands:** Located behind the thyroid gland, these glands produce parathyroid hormone (PTH):

- o **Parathyroid Hormone (PTH):** Regulates calcium levels in the blood.
  - o **Normal Range (PTH):** 10-65 pg/mL (picograms per milliliter)
  - o **Below Normal (Hypoparathyroidism):** Can cause low blood calcium (hypocalcemia), leading to muscle cramps, spasms, and tingling.
  - o **Above Normal (Hyperparathyroidism):** Can cause high blood calcium (hypercalcemia), leading to fatigue, weakness, constipation, and kidney stones.
- **Adrenal Glands:** Located on top of the kidneys, these glands produce several hormones:
  - o **Cortisol:** A stress hormone that regulates blood sugar, metabolism, and immune function.
  - o **Aldosterone:** Regulates blood pressure and electrolyte balance.
  - o **Adrenaline (Epinephrine) and Noradrenaline (Norepinephrine):** Involved in the "fight-or-flight" response.
  - o **Normal Range (Cortisol - varies by time of day):** Example: Morning: 6-23 mcg/dL
  - o **Below Normal (Adrenal Insufficiency/Addison's Disease):** Can cause fatigue, weakness, weight loss, and low blood pressure.
  - o **Above Normal (Cushing's Syndrome):** Can cause weight gain, high blood pressure, and muscle weakness.
- **Pancreas:** Located behind the stomach, the pancreas has both endocrine and digestive

functions. Its endocrine function involves producing:

- o **Insulin:** Lowers blood sugar levels by allowing glucose to enter cells.
- o **Glucagon:** Raises blood sugar levels by stimulating the liver to release stored glucose.
- o **Normal Range (Fasting Blood Glucose):** 70-100 mg/dL
- o **Above Normal (Hyperglycemia/Diabetes):** Can lead to various complications, including heart disease, kidney disease, and nerve damage.
- o **Below Normal (Hypoglycemia):** Can cause shakiness, sweating, dizziness, and confusion.

- **Ovaries (in females):** Produce:
  - o **Estrogen and Progesterone:** Regulate the menstrual cycle, pregnancy, and female sexual characteristics.
- **Testes (in males):** Produce:
  - o **Testosterone:** Regulates male sexual characteristics, muscle mass, and sperm production.

This chapter provides a detailed overview of the endocrine system. In the next chapter, we will discuss the nervous system, the body's control center. Let me know when you are ready to proceed.

Chapter 5: The Nervous System: The Body's Control Center

The nervous system is the body's primary control and communication network. It's responsible for receiving sensory information, processing that information, and coordinating responses throughout the body. This intricate system allows us to perceive the world around us, control our movements, and regulate countless internal functions.

Components of the Nervous System:

The nervous system is divided into two main parts:

- **Central Nervous System (CNS):** Consists of the brain and spinal cord. The brain is the control center, responsible for thought, memory, emotion, and voluntary movement. The spinal cord acts as a communication pathway between the brain and the rest of the body.
- **Peripheral Nervous System (PNS):** Consists of all the nerves that extend outside the CNS. It connects the CNS to the rest of the body, relaying sensory information to the CNS and carrying motor commands from the CNS to muscles and glands. The PNS is further divided into:
    - **Somatic Nervous System:** Controls voluntary movements of skeletal muscles.
    - **Autonomic Nervous System:** Regulates involuntary bodily functions such as heart rate, digestion, and breathing. The autonomic nervous system is further divided into:

- **Sympathetic Nervous System:** Prepares the body for "fight-or-flight" responses.
  - **Parasympathetic Nervous System:** Promotes "rest-and-digest" functions.

The Neuron: The Basic Unit of the Nervous System:

The neuron, or nerve cell, is the fundamental unit of the nervous system. It's responsible for transmitting electrical and chemical signals throughout the body. A neuron consists of:

- **Cell Body (Soma):** Contains the nucleus and other cellular organelles.
- **Dendrites:** Branch-like extensions that receive signals from other neurons.
- **Axon:** A long, slender extension that transmits signals away from the cell body to other neurons, muscles, or glands.
- **Synapses:** The junctions between neurons where signals are transmitted.

How Nerve Impulses are Transmitted:

Nerve impulses are transmitted through a combination of electrical and chemical signals.

1. **Electrical Signal (Action Potential):** An electrical signal travels down the axon of a neuron.
2. **Chemical Signal (Neurotransmitters):** At the synapse, the electrical signal triggers the release of neurotransmitters, chemical messengers that

diffuse across the synaptic gap and bind to receptors on the next neuron.

3. **Signal Reception:** The binding of neurotransmitters to receptors triggers an electrical signal in the receiving neuron, continuing the transmission of the nerve impulse.

Key Neurotransmitters and Their Functions:

- **Acetylcholine:** Involved in muscle contraction, memory, and learning.
- **Dopamine:** Involved in movement, motivation, reward, and pleasure.
- **Serotonin:** Involved in mood regulation, sleep, appetite, and digestion.
- **Norepinephrine (Noradrenaline):** Involved in the "fight-or-flight" response, alertness, and attention.
- **GABA (Gamma-Aminobutyric Acid):** An inhibitory neurotransmitter that helps calm the nervous system.
- **Glutamate:** An excitatory neurotransmitter involved in learning and memory.

Common Conditions Affecting the Nervous System:

- **Multiple Sclerosis (MS):** An autoimmune disease that affects the myelin sheath, the protective covering of nerve fibers, disrupting nerve signal transmission. Symptoms can include fatigue, numbness, tingling, muscle weakness, and vision problems.
- **Parkinson's Disease:** A neurodegenerative disorder that affects dopamine-producing neurons in the

brain, leading to tremors, rigidity, slow movement, and balance problems.

- **Alzheimer's Disease:** A neurodegenerative disease that causes progressive memory loss, cognitive decline, and behavioral changes.
- **Stroke:** Occurs when blood supply to the brain is interrupted, causing brain damage. Symptoms can include sudden weakness or numbness on one side of the body, difficulty speaking, and vision problems.
- **Epilepsy:** A neurological disorder characterized by recurrent seizures, which are caused by abnormal electrical activity in the brain.

This chapter provides a comprehensive overview of the nervous system. In the next chapter, we will discuss the cardiovascular system, the body's transportation network. Let me know when you're ready to proceed.

Chapter 6: The Cardiovascular System: The Body's Transportation Network

The cardiovascular system, also known as the circulatory system, is a vital network responsible for transporting blood throughout the body. This continuous flow of blood delivers oxygen, nutrients, hormones, and immune cells to tissues and organs while simultaneously removing waste products like carbon dioxide. This chapter will explore the components of this essential system and how they work together to maintain life.

Components of the Cardiovascular System:

The cardiovascular system consists of three main components:

- **The Heart:** The heart is a muscular organ that acts as a pump, propelling blood through the blood vessels. It has four chambers:
    - **Right Atrium:** Receives deoxygenated blood from the body.
    - **Right Ventricle:** Pumps deoxygenated blood to the lungs.
    - **Left Atrium:** Receives oxygenated blood from the lungs.
    - **Left Ventricle:** Pumps oxygenated blood to the rest of the body.
- **Blood Vessels:** These are the network of tubes that carry blood throughout the body. There are three main types:
    - **Arteries:** Carry oxygenated blood away from the heart to the body's tissues. The largest artery is the aorta.

- Veins: Carry deoxygenated blood back to the heart. The largest veins are the superior and inferior vena cava.
  - **Capillaries:** Tiny, thin-walled blood vessels that form a network between arteries and veins. This is where the exchange of oxygen, nutrients, and waste products occurs between the blood and the tissues.
- **Blood:** Blood is the fluid that circulates through the blood vessels, carrying oxygen, nutrients, hormones, and waste products. It consists of:
  - **Red Blood Cells (Erythrocytes):** Contain hemoglobin, which carries oxygen.
  - **White Blood Cells (Leukocytes):** Part of the immune system, fighting infection.
  - **Platelets (Thrombocytes):** Involved in blood clotting.
  - **Plasma:** The liquid portion of blood, containing water, proteins, electrolytes, and other substances.

The Cardiac Cycle:

The cardiac cycle describes the sequence of events that occur during one heartbeat. It consists of two main phases:

- **Systole:** The contraction phase, during which the heart pumps blood out into the arteries.
- **Diastole:** The relaxation phase, during which the heart fills with blood.

Blood Pressure:

Blood pressure is the force of blood against the walls of the arteries. It is measured in millimeters of mercury (mmHg) and is expressed as two numbers:

- **Systolic Pressure:** The pressure when the heart contracts (top number).
- **Diastolic Pressure:** The pressure when the heart relaxes (bottom number).
- **Normal Blood Pressure:** Around 120/80 mmHg.
- **High Blood Pressure (Hypertension):** Can increase the risk of heart disease, stroke, and kidney disease.
- **Low Blood Pressure (Hypotension):** Can cause dizziness, fainting, and fatigue.

Common Conditions Affecting the Cardiovascular System:

- **Coronary Artery Disease (CAD):** A condition in which the arteries that supply blood to the heart become narrowed or blocked, often due to plaque buildup. This can lead to chest pain (angina), heart attack, or heart failure.
- **Heart Attack (Myocardial Infarction):** Occurs when blood flow to a part of the heart is completely blocked, causing damage to the heart muscle.
- **Stroke:** Occurs when blood supply to the brain is interrupted, either by a blockage (ischemic stroke) or bleeding (hemorrhagic stroke).
- **Heart Failure:** A condition in which the heart is unable to pump enough blood to meet the body's needs.
- **Arrhythmias:** Irregular heartbeats, which can be too fast (tachycardia), too slow (bradycardia), or irregular.

Tests to Assess Cardiovascular Health:

- **Blood Pressure Measurement:** A simple and routine test to measure blood pressure.

- **Electrocardiogram (ECG/EKG):** Records the electrical activity of the heart.
- **Echocardiogram:** Uses ultrasound to create images of the heart.
- **Stress Test:** Evaluates heart function during exercise.
- **Blood Tests (Cholesterol, Lipids, etc.):** Measure levels of cholesterol and other substances in the blood that can indicate risk for heart disease.

This chapter provides a comprehensive overview of the cardiovascular system. In the next chapter, we will discuss the respiratory system, responsible for the exchange of gases. Let me know when you are ready to proceed.

Chapter 7: The Respiratory System: The Breath of Life

The respiratory system is responsible for the vital process of *gas* exchange, taking in oxygen from the air and expelling carbon dioxide, a waste product of cellular metabolism. This continuous exchange is essential for sustaining life, providing the oxygen necessary for cellular energy production and removing the carbon dioxide that would otherwise build up to toxic levels. This chapter explores the components of the respiratory system and how they work together to facilitate breathing.

Components of the Respiratory System:

The respiratory system consists of several key components:

- **Nose and Nasal Cavity:** Air enters the body through the nose and nasal cavity, where it is filtered, warmed, and humidified.
- **Pharynx (Throat):** A passageway for both air and food, connecting the nasal cavity and mouth to the larynx and esophagus.
- **Larynx (Voice Box):** Contains the vocal cords, which vibrate to produce sound.
- **Trachea (Windpipe):** A tube that carries air from the larynx to the lungs.
- **Bronchi:** The trachea branches into two main bronchi, one leading to each lung.
- **Bronchioles:** Within the lungs, the bronchi further divide into smaller and smaller tubes called bronchioles.
- **Alveoli:** Tiny air sacs at the end of the bronchioles where *gas* exchange takes place.

- **Lungs:** The primary organs of respiration, containing the bronchi, bronchioles, and alveoli.
- **Diaphragm:** A dome-shaped muscle that separates the chest cavity from the abdominal cavity and plays a crucial role in breathing.

The Process of Breathing (Ventilation):

Breathing, or ventilation, involves two main phases:

- **Inhalation (Inspiration):** The diaphragm contracts and moves downward, and the rib muscles contract, expanding the chest cavity. This creates a vacuum, drawing air into the lungs.
- **Exhalation (Expiration):** The diaphragm relaxes and moves upward, and the rib muscles relax, reducing the size of the chest cavity. This increases the pressure in the lungs, forcing air out.

Gas Exchange:

Gas exchange occurs in the alveoli. Oxygen from the inhaled air diffuses across the thin walls of the alveoli into the surrounding capillaries, where it binds to hemoglobin in red blood cells. Simultaneously, carbon dioxide from the blood diffuses from the capillaries into the alveoli to be exhaled.

Lung Capacity and Volumes:

Several measurements are used to assess lung function:

- **Tidal Volume:** The amount of air inhaled or exhaled during normal breathing.

- **Inspiratory Reserve Volume:** The additional amount of air that can be inhaled after a normal inhalation.
- **Expiratory Reserve Volume:** The additional amount of air that can be exhaled after a normal exhalation.
- **Residual Volume:** The amount of air remaining in the lungs after a maximal exhalation.
- **Vital Capacity:** The total amount of air that can be exhaled after a maximal inhalation (Tidal Volume + Inspiratory Reserve Volume + Expiratory Reserve Volume).
- **Total Lung Capacity:** The total amount of air the lungs can hold (Vital Capacity + Residual Volume).

Common Conditions Affecting the Respiratory System:

- **Asthma:** A chronic inflammatory condition of the airways that causes wheezing, shortness of breath, chest tightness, and coughing.
- **Chronic Obstructive Pulmonary Disease (COPD):** A group of lung diseases that block airflow and make it difficult to breathe, including emphysema and chronic bronchitis.
- **Pneumonia:** An infection of the lungs that causes inflammation of the alveoli.
- **Lung Cancer:** A malignant tumor that develops in the lungs.
- **Bronchitis:** Inflammation of the lining of the bronchial tubes.

Tests to Assess Respiratory Health:

- **Pulmonary Function Tests (PFTs):** Measure lung capacity and airflow.

- **Spirometry:** A common PFT that measures how much air you can inhale and exhale and how quickly you can exhale.
- **Chest X-ray:** An imaging test that can reveal abnormalities in the lungs.
- **Blood *Gas* Analysis:** Measures the levels of oxygen and carbon dioxide in the blood.

This chapter provides a detailed overview of the respiratory system. We will continue with the digestive system in the next response. Let me know when you are ready to proceed.

Chapter 8: The Digestive System: Fueling the Body

The digestive system is responsible for breaking down food into smaller molecules that the body can absorb and use for energy, growth, and repair. This complex process involves a coordinated effort of several organs, working together to ingest, digest, absorb, and eliminate waste. This chapter explores the components of the digestive system and the steps involved in digestion.

Components of the Digestive System:

The digestive system consists of the following organs:

- **Mouth:** The entry point for food. Chewing (mastication) begins the mechanical breakdown of food, and saliva, containing enzymes like amylase (which breaks down carbohydrates), starts the chemical breakdown.
- **Esophagus:** A muscular tube that connects the mouth to the stomach. Peristalsis, rhythmic muscle contractions, propels food down the esophagus.
- **Stomach:** A muscular organ that churns and mixes food with gastric juices, including hydrochloric acid and pepsin (which breaks down proteins).
- **Small Intestine:** The primary site of nutrient absorption. It is divided into three sections:
    - **Duodenum:** The first part of the small intestine, where most chemical digestion occurs with the help of enzymes from the pancreas and bile from the liver.
    - **Jejunum:** The middle part of the small intestine, where the majority of nutrient absorption takes place.

- o **Ileum:** The last part of the small intestine, where remaining nutrients and vitamin B12 are absorbed.
- **Large Intestine (Colon):** Absorbs water and electrolytes from undigested food material, forming feces.
- **Rectum and Anus:** The rectum stores feces until elimination through the anus.
- **Accessory Organs:** These organs assist in digestion but are not part of the digestive tract itself:
  - o **Liver:** Produces bile, which helps in the digestion and absorption of fats. It also plays a role in detoxification and nutrient storage.
  - o **Gallbladder:** Stores bile produced by the liver.
  - o **Pancreas:** Produces digestive enzymes (e.g., amylase, lipase, trypsin) and hormones (insulin and glucagon).

The Process of Digestion:

Digestion involves several key processes:

1. **Ingestion:** The intake of food into the mouth.
2. **Mechanical Digestion:** The physical breakdown of food into smaller pieces through chewing and churning in the stomach.
3. **Chemical Digestion:** The breakdown of food molecules by enzymes into smaller molecules that can be absorbed.
4. **Absorption:** The passage of digested nutrients from the small intestine into the bloodstream.
5. **Elimination:** The removal of undigested waste material (feces) from the body.

Enzymes Involved in Digestion:

- **Amylase:** Breaks down carbohydrates into sugars.
- **Lipase:** Breaks down fats into fatty acids and glycerol.
- **Proteases (e.g., pepsin, trypsin):** Break down proteins into amino acids.

Absorption in the Small Intestine:

The small intestine is lined with villi and microvilli, which increase the surface area for absorption. Nutrients are absorbed into the bloodstream through the walls of the small intestine and transported to the rest of the body.

Common Conditions Affecting the Digestive System:

- **Gastroesophageal Reflux Disease (GERD):** A condition in which stomach acid flows back up into the esophagus, causing heartburn.
- **Peptic Ulcers:** Sores in the lining of the stomach or duodenum.
- **Irritable Bowel Syndrome (IBS):** A common disorder that affects the large intestine, causing abdominal pain, bloating, and changes in bowel habits.
- **Inflammatory Bowel Disease (IBD):** A group of diseases that cause inflammation of the digestive tract, including Crohn's disease and ulcerative colitis.
- **Celiac Disease:** An autoimmune disorder triggered by gluten consumption, damaging the small intestine.

Tests to Assess Digestive Health:

- **Endoscopy:** A procedure in which a flexible tube with a camera is inserted into the digestive tract to visualize the lining.

- **Colonoscopy:** A specific type of endoscopy that examines the large intestine.
- **Stool Tests:** Analyze stool samples for abnormalities, such as blood or bacteria.
- **Blood Tests:** Can assess liver and pancreatic function.

This detailed explanation of the digestive system and its functions is crucial for understanding how our bodies obtain nutrients from food.

Chapter 9: The Urinary System: Maintaining Balance

The urinary system, also known as the excretory system, plays a crucial role in maintaining the body's internal environment (homeostasis). It filters waste products from the blood, regulates fluid and electrolyte balance, and helps control blood pressure. This chapter will explore the components of the urinary system and its vital functions.

Components of the Urinary System:

The urinary system consists of the following organs:

- **Kidneys:** The primary organs of the urinary system. They filter waste products from the blood and produce urine. Each kidney contains millions of microscopic filtering units called nephrons.
- **Ureters:** Two tubes that carry urine from the kidneys to the bladder.
- **Urinary Bladder:** A muscular sac that stores urine until it is eliminated from the body.
- **Urethra:** The tube that carries urine from the bladder to the outside of the body.

The Process of Urine Formation:

Urine formation involves three main processes that occur in the nephrons of the kidneys:

1. **Filtration:** Blood enters the kidneys through the renal arteries and is filtered in the glomeruli, tiny networks of capillaries within the nephrons. Water and small molecules, such as glucose, amino acids,

and waste products, are filtered out of the blood and into the nephron tubules.
2. **Reabsorption:** As the filtered fluid (filtrate) travels through the nephron tubules, essential substances, such as water, glucose, and amino acids, are reabsorbed back into the bloodstream.
3. **Secretion:** Additional waste products, such as urea, creatinine, and certain drugs, are actively secreted from the blood into the nephron tubules.

Functions of the Urinary System:

- **Waste Removal:** The primary function is to remove metabolic waste products, such as urea and creatinine, from the blood.
- **Fluid and Electrolyte Balance:** The kidneys regulate the balance of fluids and electrolytes (sodium, potassium, chloride) in the body.
- **Blood Pressure Regulation:** The kidneys help regulate blood pressure by controlling fluid volume and releasing hormones like renin.
- **Acid-Base Balance:** The kidneys help maintain the body's pH balance by regulating the excretion of hydrogen ions and bicarbonate.
- **Red Blood Cell Production:** The kidneys produce erythropoietin (EPO), a hormone that stimulates red blood cell production in the bone marrow.

Common Conditions Affecting the Urinary System:

- **Urinary Tract Infections (UTIs):** Infections of the urinary tract, usually caused by bacteria.
- **Kidney Stones:** Hard deposits of minerals and salts that form in the kidneys.

- **Kidney Disease (Chronic Kidney Disease or CKD):** A progressive loss of kidney function.
- **Kidney Failure:** A complete or near-complete loss of kidney function.
- **Incontinence:** Loss of bladder control.

Tests to Assess Urinary Health:

- **Urinalysis:** A test that analyzes a urine sample for various components, such as blood cells, protein, glucose, and bacteria.
- **Blood Tests (e.g., Creatinine, BUN):** Measure kidney function by assessing the levels of waste products in the blood.
- **Imaging Tests (e.g., Ultrasound, CT scan):** Can visualize the kidneys and other structures of the urinary system.
- **Glomerular Filtration Rate (GFR):** A measure of how well the kidneys are filtering waste products from the blood.

The skeletal system provides the structural framework for the human body, supporting soft tissues, protecting vital organs, and enabling movement. It's a dynamic system, constantly remodeling itself throughout life. This chapter explores the components of the skeletal system and its crucial functions.

Components of the Skeletal System:

The skeletal system consists of:

- **Bones:** The primary organs of the skeletal system, providing rigidity and support. There are 206 bones in the adult human body, categorized by shape:
    - **Long Bones:** Longer than they are wide (e.g., femur, humerus).
    - **Short Bones:** Roughly cube-shaped (e.g., wrist and ankle bones).
    - **Flat Bones:** Thin and flat (e.g., skull bones, ribs).
    - **Irregular Bones:** Complex shapes (e.g., vertebrae, facial bones).
- **Cartilage:** A flexible connective tissue that covers the ends of bones at joints, providing cushioning and reducing friction.
- **Ligaments:** Strong, fibrous connective tissues that connect bones to bones, stabilizing joints.
- **Tendons:** Connective tissues that connect muscles to bones, enabling movement.

Bone Structure:

Bones are composed of:

- **Compact Bone (Cortical Bone):** The dense, outer layer of bone, providing strength and rigidity.
- **Spongy Bone (Cancellous Bone):** The inner, porous layer of bone, containing red bone marrow (responsible for blood cell production) and yellow bone marrow (containing fat).
- **Periosteum:** A tough outer membrane that covers the bone surface, containing blood vessels and nerves.

Functions of the Skeletal System:

- **Support:** Provides the structural framework for the body, supporting soft tissues and organs.
- **Protection:** Protects vital organs, such as the brain (skull), heart and lungs (rib cage), and spinal cord (vertebral column).
- **Movement:** Provides attachment points for muscles, enabling movement.
- **Blood Cell Production (Hematopoiesis):** Red bone marrow produces red blood cells, white blood cells, and platelets.
- **Mineral Storage:** Bones store minerals, primarily calcium and phosphorus, which are essential for various bodily functions.

Joints:

Joints are where two or more bones meet. They allow for movement and are classified based on their structure and range of motion:

- **Fibrous Joints:** Immovable joints (e.g., sutures in the skull).
- **Cartilaginous Joints:** Allow limited movement (e.g., intervertebral discs).

- **Synovial Joints:** Freely movable joints (e.g., knee, elbow, shoulder).

Common Conditions Affecting the Skeletal System:

- **Osteoporosis:** A condition characterized by decreased bone density, making bones weak and prone to fractures.
- **Arthritis:** Inflammation of the joints, causing pain, stiffness, and swelling.
- **Fractures:** Breaks in bones, which can be caused by trauma or osteoporosis.
- **Scoliosis:** A lateral curvature of the spine.

Tests to Assess Skeletal Health:

- **X-rays:** Imaging tests that can visualize bones and detect fractures or other abnormalities.
- **Bone Density Test (DEXA Scan):** Measures bone mineral density to assess the risk of osteoporosis.
- **CT Scan and MRI:** More detailed imaging tests that can provide cross-sectional images of bones and surrounding tissues.
- **Blood Tests (e.g., Calcium, Phosphorus):** Can assess mineral levels related to bone health.

Chapter 11: The Muscular System: Enabling Movement

The muscular system is responsible for all types of body movement, from walking and running to breathing and digestion. Muscles work in conjunction with the skeletal system to produce movement, maintain posture, and generate heat. This chapter explores the different types of muscle tissue and how they function.

Types of Muscle Tissue:

There are three main types of muscle tissue in the human body:

- **Skeletal Muscle:** Attached to bones by tendons, skeletal muscle is responsible for voluntary movements. These muscles are striated (having a striped appearance) and are controlled by the somatic nervous system. Examples include the biceps, triceps, and quadriceps.
- **Smooth Muscle:** Found in the walls of internal organs, such as the stomach, intestines, blood vessels, and bladder. Smooth muscle is responsible for involuntary movements, such as digestion, blood pressure regulation, and urination. It is not striated and is controlled by the autonomic nervous system.
- **Cardiac Muscle:** Found only in the heart, cardiac muscle is responsible for pumping blood throughout the body. It is striated but is controlled involuntarily by the autonomic nervous system.

Muscle Structure:

Skeletal muscle is composed of bundles of muscle fibers (cells). Each muscle fiber contains myofibrils, which are made up of repeating units called sarcomeres. Sarcomeres contain the proteins actin and myosin, which interact to cause muscle contraction.

Muscle Contraction:

Muscle contraction occurs through a complex process involving the interaction of actin and myosin filaments within the sarcomeres. This process is triggered by nerve impulses from the nervous system.

1. A nerve impulse travels to the muscle fiber, causing the release of acetylcholine at the neuromuscular junction.
2. Acetylcholine binds to receptors on the muscle fiber, triggering an electrical signal (action potential) that spreads throughout the muscle fiber.
3. The action potential causes the release of calcium ions from the sarcoplasmic reticulum (a specialized structure within the muscle fiber).
4. Calcium ions bind to proteins on the actin filaments, allowing myosin to bind to actin.
5. Myosin heads then pull on the actin filaments, causing the sarcomere to shorten and the muscle to contract.
6. When the nerve impulse stops, calcium ions are pumped back into the sarcoplasmic reticulum, and the muscle relaxes.

Muscle Function:

- **Movement:** Muscles contract to produce movement of the skeleton, allowing us to walk, run, lift objects, and perform other physical activities.
- **Posture:** Muscles help maintain posture by constantly contracting and adjusting to keep the body upright.

- **Heat Generation:** Muscle contraction generates heat, which helps maintain body temperature.
- **Organ Function:** Smooth muscle in the walls of internal organs helps regulate various bodily functions, such as digestion, blood pressure, and urination.

Common Conditions Affecting the Muscular System:

- **Muscle Strains and Sprains:** Injuries to muscles or tendons (strains) or ligaments (sprains) caused by overstretching or tearing.
- **Muscular Dystrophy:** A group of genetic diseases that cause progressive muscle weakness and degeneration.
- **Myasthenia Gravis:** An autoimmune disease that affects the neuromuscular junction, causing muscle weakness and fatigue.
- **Fibromyalgia:** A chronic condition characterized by widespread muscle pain, fatigue, and tenderness.

Tests to Assess Muscular Health:

- **Physical Examination:** A doctor can assess muscle strength, range of motion, and reflexes.
- **Electromyography (EMG):** Measures the electrical activity of muscles.
- **Muscle Biopsy:** A small sample of muscle tissue is taken for examination under a microscope.
- **Blood Tests (e.g., Creatine Kinase):** Can detect muscle damage.

Chapter 12: The Integumentary System: The Body's Protective Shield

The integumentary system, composed of the skin, hair, nails, and associated glands, forms the body's outermost layer and acts as a vital protective barrier against the external environment. This system performs a multitude of functions, including protection, temperature regulation, sensory perception, and vitamin D synthesis. This chapter explores the components of the integumentary system and their crucial roles in maintaining health.

Components of the Integumentary System:

- **Skin:** The largest organ of the body, composed of three main layers:
    - **Epidermis:** The outermost layer, composed of stratified squamous epithelium. It provides a waterproof barrier and protects against infection. The epidermis contains specialized cells called keratinocytes, which produce keratin (a tough, fibrous protein), and melanocytes, which produce melanin (a pigment that gives skin its color and protects against UV radiation).
    - **Dermis:** The middle layer, containing connective tissue, blood vessels, nerves, hair follicles, and sweat glands. It provides strength, elasticity, and sensation to the skin.
    - **Hypodermis (Subcutaneous Layer):** The innermost layer, composed of adipose (fat) tissue and connective tissue. It insulates the

body, stores energy, and anchors the skin to underlying tissues.

- **Hair:** Composed of keratinized filaments that grow from hair follicles in the dermis. Hair provides insulation, protection, and sensory perception.
- **Nails:** Hard, keratinized plates that protect the tips of the fingers and toes.
- **Glands:**
  - **Sweat Glands:** Produce sweat, which helps regulate body temperature through evaporation. There are two main types: eccrine glands (found throughout the skin) and apocrine glands (found in the armpits and groin).
  - **Sebaceous Glands:** Produce sebum, an oily substance that lubricates the skin and hair.

Functions of the Integumentary System:

- **Protection:** The skin acts as a physical barrier against pathogens, UV radiation, and physical injury.
- **Temperature Regulation:** The skin helps regulate body temperature through sweating and by adjusting blood flow to the skin.
- **Sensory Perception:** The skin contains nerve endings that detect touch, pressure, pain, and temperature.
- **Vitamin D Synthesis:** The skin produces vitamin D when exposed to sunlight, which is essential for calcium absorption and bone health.
- **Excretion:** Small amounts of waste products are excreted through sweat.

Common Conditions Affecting the Integumentary System:

- **Acne:** A common skin condition characterized by pimples, blackheads, and whiteheads, caused by clogged hair follicles.
- **Eczema (Atopic Dermatitis):** A chronic inflammatory skin condition that causes itchy, dry, and inflamed skin.
- **Psoriasis:** A chronic autoimmune skin condition that causes red, scaly patches on the skin.
- **Skin Cancer:** The most common type of cancer, which develops in the skin cells. There are three main types: basal cell carcinoma, squamous cell carcinoma, and melanoma.
- **Infections (Bacterial, Viral, Fungal):** The skin can be susceptible to various infections caused by bacteria, viruses, or fungi.

Tests to Assess Integumentary Health:

- **Visual Examination:** A doctor can visually examine the skin, hair, and nails for abnormalities.
- **Biopsy:** A small sample of skin tissue is taken for examination under a microscope.
- **Allergy Testing:** Can identify allergens that trigger skin reactions.
- **Patch Testing:** A type of allergy testing where small amounts of allergens are applied to the skin to see if they cause a reaction.

Chapter 13: The Immune System: Defending Against Invaders

The immune system is a complex network of cells, tissues, and organs that work together to defend the body against pathogens, such as bacteria, viruses, [1] fungi, and parasites. It's a highly sophisticated system capable of recognizing and destroying foreign invaders while distinguishing them from the body's own cells. This chapter explores the components of the immune system and how they work together to protect us from disease.

Components of the Immune System:

The immune system is not confined to a single organ but is distributed throughout the body. Key components include:

- **White Blood Cells (Leukocytes):** The primary cells of the immune system. There are several types of leukocytes, each with specific functions:
  - **Phagocytes (e.g., Neutrophils, Macrophages):** Engulf and destroy pathogens through a process called phagocytosis.
  - **Lymphocytes (e.g., B cells, T cells):** Responsible for adaptive immunity, a more specific and targeted immune response.
    - **B cells:** Produce antibodies, proteins that recognize and bind to specific antigens (substances that trigger an immune response).
    - **T cells:** Several types of T cells play different roles in immunity:

- **Helper T cells:** Help activate other immune cells, including B cells and cytotoxic T cells.
          - **Cytotoxic T cells:** Directly kill infected cells.
          - **Regulatory T cells:** Help suppress the immune response to prevent autoimmunity.
- **Lymphatic System:** A network of vessels and tissues that helps circulate immune cells and filter fluids.
    - **Lymph Nodes:** Small, bean-shaped organs that filter lymph fluid and contain immune cells.
    - **Lymphatic Vessels:** Carry lymph fluid throughout the body.
    - **Spleen:** Filters blood and removes old or damaged red blood cells. It also contains immune cells.
    - **Thymus:** An organ located in the chest that is important for T cell maturation.
- **Bone Marrow:** The soft tissue inside bones where blood cells, including immune cells, are produced.
- **Mucous Membranes:** The linings of the respiratory, digestive, and urogenital tracts, which produce mucus that traps pathogens.
- **Skin:** As discussed in the previous chapter, the skin acts as a physical barrier against infection.

Types of Immunity:

- **Innate Immunity:** The body's first line of defense, providing a rapid, non-specific response to pathogens. It includes physical barriers (skin, mucous membranes), phagocytes, and natural killer cells.

- **Adaptive Immunity:** A more specific and targeted immune response that develops after exposure to a pathogen. It involves lymphocytes (B cells and T cells) and the production of antibodies.

The Immune Response:

When a pathogen enters the body, the immune system mounts a complex response:

1. **Recognition:** Immune cells recognize the pathogen as foreign.
2. **Activation:** Immune cells are activated and begin to multiply.
3. **Attack:** Immune cells attack and destroy the pathogen.
4. **Memory:** The immune system remembers the pathogen, providing long-lasting immunity.

Common Conditions Affecting the Immune System:

- **Autoimmune Diseases:** Conditions in which the immune system mistakenly attacks the body's own cells, such as rheumatoid arthritis, lupus, and type 1 diabetes.
- **Immunodeficiency Disorders:** Conditions in which the immune system is weakened, making individuals more susceptible to infections, such as HIV/AIDS.
- **Allergies:** An exaggerated immune response to harmless substances, such as pollen, dust mites, or food.

Tests to Assess Immune Health:

- **Complete Blood Count (CBC):** Measures the number of different types of blood cells, including white blood cells.
- **Immunoglobulin Levels:** Measure the levels of antibodies in the blood.
- **Allergy Testing:** Can identify allergens that trigger immune responses.

Chapter 14: The Reproductive System: The Cycle of Life

The reproductive system is responsible for the continuation of the human species through sexual reproduction. It consists of organs and structures that produce gametes (sex cells—sperm in males and eggs in females) and facilitate fertilization and development. This chapter will explore the male and female reproductive systems and their respective functions.

The Male Reproductive System:

The primary function of the male reproductive system is to produce, store, and transport sperm. It consists of:

- **Testes (Testicles):** The primary male reproductive organs, located in the scrotum (a pouch of skin outside the body). The testes produce sperm (spermatogenesis) and testosterone, the primary male sex hormone.
- **Epididymis:** A coiled tube located on the back of each testis where sperm mature and are stored.
- **Vas Deferens:** A tube that carries sperm from the epididymis to the urethra.
- **Seminal Vesicles:** Glands that produce a fluid that contributes to semen.
- **Prostate Gland:** A gland that produces a fluid that also contributes to semen.
- **Bulbourethral Glands (Cowper's Glands):** Glands that produce a lubricating fluid that is released before ejaculation.
- **Urethra:** The tube that carries both urine and semen out of the body (though not at the same time).
- **Penis:** The external male reproductive organ.

Spermatogenesis:

Spermatogenesis, the production of sperm, occurs in the seminiferous tubules within the testes. This process is stimulated by follicle-stimulating hormone (FSH) and testosterone.

The Female Reproductive System:

The primary functions of the female reproductive system are to produce eggs (ova), provide a site for fertilization and development of a fetus, and give birth. It consists of:

- **Ovaries:** The primary female reproductive organs, located in the pelvic cavity. The ovaries produce eggs (oogenesis) and female sex hormones (estrogen and progesterone).
- **Fallopian Tubes (Oviducts):** Tubes that carry eggs from the ovaries to the uterus. Fertilization typically occurs in the fallopian tubes.
- **Uterus (Womb):** A muscular organ where a fertilized egg implants and develops [1] during pregnancy.

1. brainly.in

- **Cervix:** The lower part of the uterus that connects to the vagina.
- **Vagina:** A muscular canal that connects the cervix to the outside of the body.
- **Vulva:** The external female genitalia, including the labia, clitoris, and vaginal opening.

Oogenesis and the Menstrual Cycle:

Oogenesis, the production of eggs, begins before birth but is completed after puberty with each menstrual cycle. The menstrual cycle is a monthly cycle of hormonal changes that prepares the uterus for pregnancy. It involves:

1. **Follicular Phase:** FSH stimulates the development of follicles in the ovaries, each containing an egg.
2. **Ovulation:** LH surge triggers the release of an egg from the ovary.
3. **Luteal Phase:** The ruptured follicle becomes the corpus luteum, which produces progesterone.
4. **Menstruation:** If fertilization does not occur, the corpus luteum degenerates, and the uterine lining is shed (menstruation).

Fertilization and Pregnancy:

If sperm fertilizes an egg in the fallopian tube, the fertilized egg (zygote) travels to the uterus and implants in the uterine lining. Pregnancy then begins, and the developing embryo/fetus receives nourishment and oxygen from the mother through the placenta.

Common Conditions Affecting the Reproductive System:

- **Infertility:** The inability to conceive after a certain period of time.
- **Sexually Transmitted Infections (STIs):** Infections transmitted through sexual contact.
- **Endometriosis (Females):** A condition in which tissue similar to the uterine lining grows outside the uterus.
- **Polycystic Ovary Syndrome (PCOS) (Females):** A hormonal disorder that can cause irregular periods, ovarian cysts, and infertility.
- **Prostate Cancer (Males):** A cancer that develops in the prostate gland.

Tests to Assess Reproductive Health:

- **Physical Examination:** A doctor can perform a physical examination of the reproductive organs.
- **Hormone Testing:** Measures levels of reproductive hormones in the blood.
- **Semen Analysis (Males):** Evaluates sperm count, motility, and morphology.
- **Ultrasound:** Can visualize the reproductive organs.

Part 3

Chapter 15: Blood Tests: A Window into Your Health

Blood tests are among the most common diagnostic tools used in medicine. They provide valuable information about various aspects of your health, from organ function and blood cell counts to cholesterol levels and hormone levels. Understanding what these tests measure and what the results mean can empower you to take a more active role in managing your health. This chapter will explore some of the most common blood tests and their significance.

What is Blood?

Before diving into specific tests, let's briefly recap the composition of blood:

- **Plasma:** The liquid component of blood, consisting mostly of water but also containing proteins (like albumin, globulins, and clotting factors), electrolytes (like sodium, potassium, and chloride), hormones, nutrients, and waste products.
- **Red Blood Cells (Erythrocytes):** Responsible for transporting oxygen from the lungs to the body's tissues. They contain hemoglobin, an iron-rich protein that binds to oxygen.
- **White Blood Cells (Leukocytes):** Part of the immune system, defending the body against infection. There are several types of white blood cells, each with specific functions (e.g., neutrophils, lymphocytes, monocytes, eosinophils, basophils).
- **Platelets (Thrombocytes):** Small cell fragments involved in blood clotting.

Common Blood Tests and Their Significance:

- **Complete Blood Count (CBC):** This is a very common test that provides a comprehensive overview of your blood cells:
  - **Red Blood Cell Count (RBC):** Measures the number of red blood cells.
    - **Below Normal (Anemia):** Can indicate iron deficiency, vitamin deficiencies, blood loss, or other conditions.
    - **Above Normal (Polycythemia):** Can be caused by dehydration, certain medical conditions, or smoking.
  - **Hemoglobin (Hb):** Measures the amount of hemoglobin in the blood.
    - **Below Normal:** Indicates anemia.
    - **Above Normal:** Can indicate polycythemia.
  - **Hematocrit (Hct):** Measures the percentage of red blood cells in the blood.
    - **Below Normal:** Indicates anemia.
    - **Above Normal:** Can indicate dehydration or polycythemia.
  - **White Blood Cell Count (WBC):** Measures the number of white blood cells.
    - **Below Normal (Leukopenia):** Can indicate infection, autoimmune disorders, or certain medications.
    - **Above Normal (Leukocytosis):** Can indicate infection, inflammation, or certain cancers.
  - **Platelet Count:** Measures the number of platelets.

- - **Below Normal (Thrombocytopenia):** Can increase the risk of bleeding.
    - **Above Normal (Thrombocytosis):** Can increase the risk of blood clots.
- **Basic Metabolic Panel (BMP):** Measures several key substances in the blood, providing information about kidney function, electrolyte balance, blood sugar, and acid-base balance:
  - **Glucose:** Measures blood sugar levels.
    - **Above Normal (Hyperglycemia):** Can indicate diabetes or prediabetes.
    - **Below Normal (Hypoglycemia):** Can be caused by various factors, including diabetes medications, skipping meals, or certain medical conditions.
  - **Electrolytes (Sodium, Potassium, Chloride, Bicarbonate):** Measure the levels of these important minerals. Imbalances can indicate dehydration, kidney problems, or other conditions.
  - **Kidney Function Tests (Creatinine, BUN - Blood Urea Nitrogen):** Measure how well the kidneys are filtering waste products from the blood. Elevated levels can indicate kidney disease.
- **Comprehensive Metabolic Panel (CMP):** Includes all the tests in the BMP plus liver function tests:
  - **Liver Function Tests (ALT, AST, ALP, Bilirubin):** Measure liver enzymes and bilirubin, which can indicate liver damage or disease.
- **Lipid Panel:** Measures cholesterol and triglycerides, which are important risk factors for heart disease:

- **Total Cholesterol:**
  - **LDL Cholesterol ("Bad" Cholesterol):** High levels increase the risk of heart disease.
  - **HDL Cholesterol ("Good" Cholesterol):** High levels are protective against heart disease.
  - **Triglycerides:** High levels can increase the risk of heart disease.
- **Thyroid Panel:** Measures thyroid hormone levels to assess thyroid function (as discussed in Chapter 4).
- **C-Reactive Protein (CRP):** Measures inflammation in the body. Elevated levels can indicate infection, inflammation, or other conditions.

Chapter 16: Urine Tests: Analyzing Waste Products

Urine tests, or urinalysis, analyze the composition of urine to detect and manage a wide range of health conditions. Because the kidneys filter waste products from the blood and excrete them in urine, analyzing urine can provide valuable insights into kidney function, metabolic processes, and the presence of infections. This chapter will explore different types of urine tests and their clinical significance.

What is Urine?

Urine is a liquid waste product produced by the kidneys. It primarily consists of water but also contains various dissolved substances, including:

- **Urea:** A waste product of protein metabolism.
- **Creatinine:** A waste product of muscle metabolism.
- **Electrolytes:** Such as sodium, potassium, and chloride.
- **Other metabolic waste products:** Such as uric acid.

Types of Urine Tests:

- **Routine Urinalysis:** This is the most common type of urine test and involves a visual examination, chemical analysis, and microscopic examination of the urine:
  - **Visual Examination:** Assesses the urine's color, clarity (clear or cloudy), and odor.
  - **Chemical Analysis (Dipstick Test):** Uses a dipstick with chemical pads that react to various substances in the urine, providing quick results for:
    - **pH:** Measures the acidity or alkalinity of the urine.

- **Specific Gravity:** Measures the concentration of particles in the urine.
        - **Protein:** Detects the presence of protein in the urine, which can indicate kidney damage.
        - **Glucose:** Detects the presence of glucose in the urine, which can indicate diabetes.
        - **Ketones:** Detects the presence of ketones in the urine, which can indicate uncontrolled diabetes or starvation.
        - **Blood (Hemoglobin):** Detects the presence of blood in the urine, which can indicate kidney stones, infection, or other conditions.
        - **Leukocyte Esterase:** Detects the presence of white blood cells in the urine, which can indicate a urinary tract infection (UTI).
        - **Nitrite:** Detects the presence of nitrites in the urine, which can also indicate a UTI.
    - **Microscopic Examination:** Examines the urine under a microscope to identify:
        - **Red Blood Cells:** Can indicate kidney stones, infection, or other conditions.
        - **White Blood Cells:** Can indicate a UTI or other infections.
        - **Bacteria:** Can indicate a UTI.
        - **Crystals:** Can indicate kidney stones or other metabolic disorders.
        - **Casts:** Microscopic cylindrical structures that can indicate kidney disease.

- **Urine Culture:** This test is used to identify the specific type of bacteria causing a UTI. A urine sample is placed in a culture medium to allow bacteria to grow, and then the bacteria are identified.
- **24-Hour Urine Collection:** This test involves collecting all urine produced over a 24-hour period. It is used to measure the amount of certain substances in the urine, such as protein, creatinine, or calcium, and can provide more accurate assessments of kidney function or hormone levels.

Clinical Significance of Urine Test Results:

- **Changes in Color:** Can be caused by dehydration (dark yellow), certain foods or medications, or blood in the urine (red or pink).
- **Changes in Clarity:** Cloudy urine can indicate infection or the presence of crystals.
- **Abnormal pH:** Can indicate kidney or respiratory problems.
- **Proteinuria (Protein in Urine):** Can indicate kidney damage or other conditions.
- **Glucosuria (Glucose in Urine):** Can indicate diabetes.
- **Ketonuria (Ketones in Urine):** Can indicate uncontrolled diabetes, starvation, or a high-fat diet.
- **Hematuria (Blood in Urine):** Can indicate kidney stones, infection, bladder cancer, or other conditions.
- **Pyuria (White Blood Cells in Urine):** Indicates infection, typically a UTI.
- **Bacteria in Urine:** Indicates a UTI.

Urine tests are valuable tools for diagnosing and monitoring a variety of health conditions. They are relatively non-invasive and can provide important information about the body's internal environment.

Chapter 17: Hormone Testing: Measuring the Body's Chemical Messengers

Hormones, as discussed in Chapter 4, are chemical messengers that regulate a wide range of bodily functions. Hormone testing plays a crucial role in diagnosing and managing conditions related to hormonal imbalances. These tests measure the levels of specific hormones in the blood, urine, or saliva, providing valuable insights into the function of the endocrine system. This chapter will explore various hormone tests and their clinical significance.

Types of Hormone Tests and Their Significance:

- **Thyroid Hormone Tests:** These tests assess the function of the thyroid gland:
    - **Thyroid-Stimulating Hormone (TSH):** Measures the level of TSH, a hormone produced by the pituitary gland that stimulates the thyroid to produce thyroid hormones. [1] TSH is often the first test performed to assess thyroid function.
        - **High TSH, Low T4/T3:** Suggests hypothyroidism (underactive thyroid).
        - **Low TSH, High T4/T3:** Suggests hyperthyroidism (overactive
    - **Thyroxine (T4):** Measures the level of T4, the main hormone produced by the thyroid gland.
    - **Triiodothyronine (T3):** Measures the level of T3, a more active form of thyroid hormone.
    - **Free T4 and Free T3:** Measure the levels of T4 and T3 that are not bound to proteins in

the blood and are therefore available to exert their effects on the body. These are often considered more accurate measures of thyroid function.

- **Reproductive Hormone Tests:** These tests assess the function of the reproductive organs:
  - **Follicle-Stimulating Hormone (FSH):** In females, FSH stimulates the development of follicles in the ovaries. In males, FSH stimulates sperm production.
  - **Luteinizing Hormone (LH):** In females, LH triggers ovulation. In males, LH stimulates testosterone production.
  - **Estradiol (E2):** The primary female sex hormone.
  - **Progesterone:** A female sex hormone involved in the menstrual cycle and pregnancy.
  - **Testosterone:** The primary male sex hormone.
- **Adrenal Hormone Tests:** These tests assess the function of the adrenal glands:
  - **Cortisol:** Measures the level of cortisol, a stress hormone. Cortisol levels typically follow a diurnal rhythm, with higher levels in the morning and lower levels in the evening. Testing may involve multiple samples taken throughout the day.
  - **ACTH (Adrenocorticotropic Hormone):** Measures the level of ACTH, a hormone produced by the pituitary gland that stimulates the adrenal glands to produce cortisol.

- o **Aldosterone:** Measures the level of aldosterone, a hormone that regulates blood pressure and electrolyte balance.
- **Growth Hormone (GH) and Insulin-like Growth Factor 1 (IGF-1):** These tests assess growth hormone production:
    - o **Growth Hormone (GH):** GH levels fluctuate throughout the day, so a single measurement is not always informative. Stimulation or suppression tests may be performed.
    - o **IGF-1:** IGF-1 is a hormone produced by the liver in response to GH. It provides a more stable measure of GH activity.
- **Parathyroid Hormone (PTH):** Measures the level of PTH, a hormone that regulates calcium levels in the blood.

Methods of Hormone Testing:

- **Blood Tests:** The most common method for measuring hormone levels.
- **Urine Tests:** Can be used to measure certain hormones or hormone metabolites.
- **Saliva Tests:** Can be used to measure certain hormones, such as cortisol.

Interpreting Hormone Test Results:

It is crucial to interpret hormone test results in the context of a person's medical history, symptoms, and other test results. Reference ranges can vary slightly between laboratories, so it's important to refer to the specific lab's reference range when interpreting results. A healthcare professional is best equipped to interpret hormone test results and determine the appropriate course of action.

Chapter 18: Imaging Techniques: Seeing Inside the Body

Imaging techniques are essential tools in modern medicine, allowing healthcare professionals to visualize the internal structures of the body without the need for invasive surgery. These techniques play a crucial role in diagnosing a wide range of conditions, from broken bones and tumors to internal organ damage and blood vessel abnormalities. This chapter will explore several common imaging techniques and their applications.

Types of Imaging Techniques:

- **X-ray:** X-rays use electromagnetic radiation to create images of dense structures, such as bones. They are commonly used to:
    - Detect fractures and other bone injuries.
    - Identify foreign objects.
    - Diagnose lung conditions, such as pneumonia and lung cancer.
    - Examine the teeth.
- **Computed Tomography (CT) Scan:** CT scans use X-rays taken from multiple angles to create cross-sectional images of the body. They provide more detailed images than traditional X-rays and are used to:
    - Visualize internal organs, such as the brain, lungs, liver, and kidneys.
    - Detect tumors, infections, and internal bleeding.
    - Guide biopsies and other minimally invasive procedures.
- **Magnetic Resonance Imaging (MRI):** MRI uses strong magnetic fields and radio waves to create

detailed images of the body's soft tissues, including organs, muscles, ligaments, and the brain. It is used to:

- o Diagnose brain and spinal cord disorders.
- o Evaluate joint injuries.
- o Detect tumors and other abnormalities in soft tissues.

- **Ultrasound:** Ultrasound uses high-frequency sound waves to create images of internal organs and tissues. It is a safe and non-invasive technique commonly used to:
  - o Monitor fetal development during pregnancy.
  - o Examine the heart, liver, gallbladder, kidneys, and other organs.
  - o Guide biopsies and other procedures.

- **Positron Emission Tomography (PET) Scan:** PET scans use a radioactive tracer to detect metabolic activity in tissues and organs. They are often used to:
  - o Detect cancer and assess its spread.
  - o Evaluate brain function.
  - o Assess heart function.

How Imaging Techniques Work (Simplified):

- **X-ray:** X-rays pass through soft tissues but are absorbed by denser tissues like bone, creating a shadow image on a detector.
- **CT Scan:** X-ray beams rotate around the patient, and detectors measure the amount of radiation absorbed by different tissues. A computer then reconstructs these measurements into cross-sectional images.

- **MRI:** Strong magnetic fields align the protons in the body's water molecules. Radio waves are then used to briefly disrupt this alignment, and the signals emitted by the protons as they realign are detected and used to create images.
- **Ultrasound:** High-frequency sound waves are emitted from a transducer and bounce back off tissues and organs. The echoes are then processed to create images.
- **PET Scan:** A radioactive tracer is injected into the body and accumulates in areas with high metabolic activity, such as cancer cells. The scanner detects the radiation emitted by the tracer to create images.

Safety Considerations:

- **Radiation Exposure:** X-rays and CT scans use ionizing radiation, which carries a small risk of cancer. However, the benefits of these scans usually outweigh the risks. MRI and ultrasound do not use ionizing radiation and are considered safe. PET scans involve exposure to a small amount of radioactive material.
- **Contrast Dyes:** Sometimes, contrast dyes are used in CT and MRI scans to enhance the visibility of certain tissues or organs. These dyes can cause allergic reactions in some individuals.

Imaging techniques have revolutionized medical diagnosis and treatment, providing invaluable insights into the inner workings of the human body.

Conclusion: Taking Charge of Your Health

This book, "The Body Blueprint," has taken you on a journey through the intricate landscape of the human body, exploring its elemental composition, complex systems, and the various tests used to assess its health. From the microscopic world of cells and molecules to the coordinated functions of organ systems, you've gained a deeper understanding of how your body works and the factors that influence its well-being.

The goal of this book has not been to turn you into a medical expert, but rather to empower you with knowledge. By understanding the building blocks of life (minerals, vitamins, proteins, and carbohydrates), the functions of your body's systems (endocrine, nervous, cardiovascular, respiratory, digestive, urinary, skeletal, muscular, integumentary, immune, and reproductive), and the insights provided by various medical tests, you can take a more proactive and informed approach to your health.

Key Takeaways:

- **Your body is a complex and interconnected system:** Each part plays a vital role in maintaining overall health.
- **Nutrition is essential:** A balanced diet rich in essential nutrients is crucial for optimal bodily function.
- **Understanding your body's signals is key:** Pay attention to changes in your body and consult with healthcare professionals when necessary.
- **Medical tests provide valuable insights:** Understanding what these tests measure and what

the results mean can empower you to make informed decisions about your health.

- **Proactive health management is crucial:** Taking steps to maintain your health through diet, exercise, and regular checkups can significantly improve your well-being.

Moving Forward

The knowledge you've gained from this book is a starting point. Continue to learn about your body and stay informed about the latest health information. Here are some steps you can take to further enhance your self-awareness and take charge of your health:

- **Establish a relationship with a trusted healthcare provider:** Regular checkups and open communication with your doctor are essential for preventive care and early detection of health problems.
- **Adopt a healthy lifestyle:** This includes eating a balanced diet, engaging in regular physical activity, getting enough sleep, and managing stress.
- **Learn to recognize your body's signals:** Pay attention to any changes in your body and consult with a healthcare professional if you have concerns.
- **Utilize reliable health resources:** Seek information from reputable sources, such as government health websites, medical organizations, and peer-reviewed journals.
- **Be an advocate for your own health:** Ask questions, seek second opinions if necessary, and actively participate in your healthcare decisions.

A Final Thought

"Know thyself," as the ancient Greek aphorism states, is a cornerstone of wisdom. By understanding your body—its composition, its functions, and its signals—you are empowered to make choices that support your health and well-being. This knowledge is your personal "Body Blueprint," a guide to living a healthier, more fulfilling life.

Appendix: Glossary of Medical Terms

- **Acid-Base Balance:** The balance between acids and bases in the body's fluids, crucial for maintaining proper pH.
- **Acetylcholine:** A neurotransmitter involved in muscle contraction, memory, and learning.
- **Actin:** A protein involved in muscle contraction.
- **Action Potential:** An electrical signal that travels down a nerve cell.
- **Adipose Tissue:** Fat tissue.
- **Adrenal Glands:** Endocrine glands located on top of the kidneys that produce hormones like cortisol and adrenaline.
- **Aldosterone:** A hormone produced by the adrenal glands that regulates blood pressure and electrolyte balance.
- **Alveoli:** Tiny air sacs in the lungs where *gas* exchange takes place.
- **Amino Acids:** The building blocks of proteins.
- **Amylase:** An enzyme that breaks down carbohydrates.
- **Anemia:** A condition characterized by a deficiency of red blood cells or hemoglobin.
- **Antibodies:** Proteins produced by B cells that recognize and bind to specific antigens.
- **Antigen:** A substance that triggers an immune response.
- **Aorta:** The largest artery in the body.
- **Arrhythmias:** Irregular heartbeats.
- **Arteries:** Blood vessels that carry blood away from the heart.
- **ATP (Adenosine Triphosphate):** The body's primary energy currency.

- **Atrium (plural: Atria):** One of the upper chambers of the heart.
- **Autonomic Nervous System:** The part of the nervous system that regulates involuntary bodily functions.
- **B Cells:** Lymphocytes that produce antibodies.
- **Bilirubin:** A waste product produced by the breakdown of heme (a component of hemoglobin).
- **Blood Urea Nitrogen (BUN):** A measure of kidney function.
- **Bronchi:** The two main branches of the trachea that lead to the lungs.
- **Bronchioles:** Smaller branches of the bronchi within the lungs.
- **Calcium (Ca):** A mineral essential for bone health, muscle contraction, nerve transmission, and blood clotting.
- **Capillaries:** Tiny blood vessels where the exchange of oxygen, nutrients, and waste products occurs.
- **Carbohydrates:** The body's primary source of energy, classified as simple or complex.
- **Cardiac Muscle:** The muscle tissue of the heart.
- **Cartilage:** A flexible connective tissue found in joints and other parts of the body.
- **Cell Membrane:** The outer boundary of a cell.
- **Central Nervous System (CNS):** The brain and spinal cord.
- **Cervix:** The lower part of the uterus.
- **Chloride (Cl):** An electrolyte involved in fluid balance, acid-base balance, and digestion.
- **Cholesterol:** A lipid (fat-like substance) found in the blood.
- **Compact Bone:** The dense, outer layer of bone.

- **Connective Tissue:** Tissue that provides support and structure to other tissues and organs.
- **Copper (Cu):** A trace mineral involved in iron metabolism and enzyme activity.
- **Cortisol:** A stress hormone produced by the adrenal glands.
- **Creatinine:** A waste product of muscle metabolism.
- **Cytoplasm:** The gel-like substance inside a cell.
- **Dendrites:** Branch-like extensions of a neuron that receive signals.
- **Dermis:** The middle layer of the skin.
- **Diaphragm:** A muscle that separates the chest cavity from the abdominal cavity and is involved in breathing.
- **Digestion:** The process of breaking down food into smaller molecules.
- **DNA (Deoxyribonucleic Acid):** The genetic material of cells.
- **Electrolytes:** Minerals that have an electrical charge and are important for fluid balance, nerve and muscle function, and other bodily processes.
- **Endocrine System:** The system of glands that produce and secrete hormones.
- **Enzymes:** Proteins that catalyze biochemical reactions.
- **Epidermis:** The outermost layer of the skin.
- **Epithelial Tissue:** Tissue that covers the body's surfaces and lines organs and cavities.
- **Esophagus:** The tube that connects the mouth to the stomach.
- **Estrogen:** A primary female sex hormone.
- **Exhalation (Expiration):** The process of breathing out.

- **Fallopian Tubes (Oviducts):** Tubes that carry eggs from the ovaries to the uterus.
- **Folate/Folic Acid (Vitamin B9):** A vitamin crucial for cell growth and division.
- **Follicle-Stimulating Hormone (FSH):** A hormone that stimulates the development of follicles in the ovaries and sperm production in males.
- **Gallbladder:** An organ that stores bile produced by the liver.
- **GABA (Gamma-Aminobutyric Acid):** An inhibitory neurotransmitter.
- **Glucagon:** A hormone produced by the pancreas that raises blood sugar levels.
- **Glutamate:** An excitatory neurotransmitter.
- **Hemoglobin (Hb):** The protein in red blood cells that carries oxygen.
- **Hematocrit (Hct):** The percentage of red blood cells in the blood.
- **Hormones:** Chemical messengers produced by endocrine glands.
- **Hypodermis (Subcutaneous Layer):** The innermost layer of the skin.
- **Hypothalamus:** A region of the brain that controls the pituitary gland and links the nervous system to
- **Inhalation (Inspiration):** The process of breathing in.
- **Insulin:** A hormone produced by the pancreas that lowers blood sugar levels.
- **Integumentary System:** The skin, hair, nails, and associated glands.
- **Iodine (I):** A trace mineral essential for thyroid hormone production.
- **Iron (Fe):** A trace mineral essential for oxygen transport.

- **Kidneys:** The primary organs of the urinary system that filter waste products from the blood.
- **Larynx:** The voice box.
- **Large Intestine (Colon):** The part of the digestive system that absorbs water and electrolytes from undigested food.
- **Leukocytes (White Blood Cells):** Cells of the immune system.
- **Ligaments:** Connective tissues that connect bones to bones.
- **Lipase:** An enzyme that breaks down fats.
- **Lipids:** Fats.
- **Liver:** An organ that produces bile and performs other important functions.
- **Lungs:** The primary organs of respiration.
- **Luteinizing Hormone (LH):** A hormone that triggers ovulation in females and stimulates testosterone production in males.
- **Lymphatic System:** A network of vessels and tissues that helps circulate immune cells and filter fluids.
- **Lymphocytes:** A type of white blood cell, including B cells and T cells.
- **Magnesium (Mg):** A mineral involved in numerous bodily functions, including muscle and nerve function.
- **Manganese (Mn):** A trace mineral involved in bone formation and metabolism.
- **Melanin:** A pigment that gives skin its color.
- **Minerals:** Naturally occurring inorganic substances essential for health.
- **Molybdenum (Mo):** A trace mineral that is a cofactor for several enzymes.
- **Muscular System:** The system of muscles that enables movement.

- **Myelin Sheath:** A protective covering around nerve fibers.
- **Myosin:** A protein involved in muscle contraction.
- **Nails:** Hard, keratinized plates that protect the tips of the fingers and toes.
- **Nasal Cavity:** The space inside the nose.
- **Nephrons:** The filtering units of the kidneys.
- **Nerve Impulse:** An electrical signal transmitted by neurons.
- **Nervous System:** The body's control and communication network, consisting of the central and peripheral nervous systems.
- **Neurons:** Nerve cells.
- **Neurotransmitters:** Chemical messengers that transmit signals between neurons.
- **Norepinephrine (Noradrenaline):** A neurotransmitter involved in the "fight-or-flight" response.
- **Ovaries:** The primary female reproductive organs that produce eggs and female sex hormones.
- **Oxytocin:** A hormone involved in uterine contractions and milk ejection.
- **Pancreas:** An organ that produces digestive enzymes and hormones (insulin and glucagon).
- **Parathyroid Glands:** Glands located behind the thyroid that produce parathyroid hormone.
- **Parathyroid Hormone (PTH):** A hormone that regulates calcium levels in the blood.
- **Pathogens:** Disease-causing microorganisms, such as bacteria, viruses, fungi, and parasites
- **Penis:** The external male reproductive organ.
- **Pepsin:** An enzyme that breaks down proteins in the stomach.

- **Peripheral Nervous System (PNS):** All the nerves outside the brain and spinal cord.
- **Periosteum:** The outer membrane that covers bone.
- **Peristalsis:** Rhythmic muscle contractions that propel food through the digestive tract.
- **pH:** A measure of acidity or alkalinity.
- **Phagocytes:** Immune cells that engulf and destroy pathogens.
- **Pharynx:** The throat.
- **Phosphorus (P):** A mineral essential for bone health, energy production, and other functions.
- **Pituitary Gland:** The "master gland" that controls other endocrine glands.
- **Plasma:** The liquid portion of blood.
- **Platelets (Thrombocytes):** Blood cell fragments involved in blood clotting.
- **Potassium (K):** An electrolyte essential for muscle and nerve function.
- **Progesterone:** A female sex hormone.
- **Proteases:** Enzymes that break down proteins.
- **Proteins:** Large molecules made up of amino acids, essential for building and repairing tissues.
- **Red Blood Cells (Erythrocytes):** Blood cells that carry oxygen.
- **Rectum:** The final section of the large intestine.
- **Reproductive System:** The system of organs involved in reproduction.
- **Residual Volume:** The amount of air remaining in the lungs after maximal exhalation.
- **Respiratory System:** The system of organs involved in *gas* exchange.

- **Riboflavin (Vitamin B2):** A B vitamin involved in energy metabolism.
- **RNA (Ribonucleic Acid):** A molecule involved in protein synthesis.
- **Saliva:** Fluid produced in the mouth that contains enzymes for digestion.
- **Sarcomeres:** The repeating units within muscle fibers that are responsible for muscle contraction.
- **Sebaceous Glands:** Glands in the skin that produce sebum (*oil*).
- **Sebum:** An oily substance produced by sebaceous glands.
- **Selenium (Se):** A trace mineral involved in antioxidant defense and thyroid hormone metabolism.
- **Semen:** The fluid containing sperm.
- **Seminal Vesicles:** Glands that contribute fluid to semen.
- **Serotonin:** A neurotransmitter involved in mood regulation, sleep, and appetite.
- **Skeletal Muscle:** Muscle tissue attached to bones, responsible for voluntary movement.
- **Skeletal System:** The system of bones, cartilage, ligaments, and tendons that provides support and structure to the body.
- **Skin:** The outer protective layer of the body.
- **Small Intestine:** The primary site of nutrient absorption in the digestive system.
- **Smooth Muscle:** Muscle tissue found in the walls of internal organs, responsible for involuntary movement.

- **Sodium (Na):** An electrolyte involved in fluid balance, nerve and muscle function, and blood pressure regulation.
- **Spongy Bone:** The inner, porous layer of bone.
- **Spleen:** An organ that filters blood and contains immune cells.
- **Stomach:** A muscular organ that churns and mixes food with gastric juices.
- **Synapses:** The junctions between neurons where signals are transmitted.
- **T Cells:** Lymphocytes involved in cell-mediated immunity.
- **T3 (Triiodothyronine):** A thyroid hormone.
- **T4 (Thyroxine):** A thyroid hormone.
- **Tendons:** Connective tissues that connect muscles to bones.
- **Testes (Testicles):** The primary male reproductive organs that produce sperm and testosterone.
- **Testosterone:** The primary male sex hormone.
- **Thiamine (Vitamin B1):** A B vitamin involved in energy metabolism.
- **Thrombocytes (Platelets):** Blood cell fragments involved in blood clotting.
- **Thymus:** An organ important for T cell maturation.
- **Thyroid Gland:** An endocrine gland in the neck that produces thyroid hormones.
- **Trachea:** The windpipe.
- **Triglycerides:** A type of fat found in the blood.
- **Urea:** A waste product of protein metabolism.
- **Ureters:** Tubes that carry urine from the kidneys to the bladder.
- **Urethra:** The tube that carries urine out of the body.

- **Urinary Bladder:** An organ that stores urine.
- **Urinary System:** The system of organs involved in filtering waste from the blood and producing urine.
- **Urine:** Liquid waste product produced by the kidneys.
- **Vagina:** The muscular canal that connects the cervix to the outside of the female body.
- **Vas Deferens:** A tube that carries sperm from the epididymis to the urethra.
- **Veins:** Blood vessels that carry blood back to the heart.
- **Ventricle:** One of the lower chambers of the heart.
- **Villi:** Finger-like projections in the small intestine that increase surface area for absorption.
- **Vitamins:** Organic compounds essential for various bodily functions.
- **Vulva:** The external female genitalia.
- **White Blood Cells (Leukocytes):** Cells of the immune system.
- **Zinc (Zn):** A trace mineral involved in immune function, cell growth, and enzyme activity.